The VAJJ. This book contains divine information on

maintaining perfect yoni (vagina) health by total yoni honor.

Here I will guide you in making friends with your deepest

mystery and teach you how to master your flows and always

maintain clear communication with your most delicate and

powerful place. The Vajjina. Best Regards love Christa Luv.

The Stories we Hear & The stories we Experience.

Mastering the mystery of being. He said to me last night. "

You are cramping because you want to make a baby. " When

we are in love your body wants to make a baby." Hmm.. I found

it sweet Arle said this to me. Just noting his intuitive

observation gave me the feeling of ease. Suddenly my cramps

subsided and I thought, " Your right I want to make a baby." It

was not just romantic talk, it was a sound the alarm statement.

We are designed in this divine way and there is always a

creative energy in us Hungry to get out and be heard and

seen. I loved how my lover comforted me last night by this

statement. And because I was relaxed and on my moon I was

able to be open and feel the truth and love of his words. " You

ache because when you love you want to make a baby. You

ache because you long for that fulfillment." Hmm.. I am now

alone at home after Arle has brought me home and I realize I

am still resonating with his shared intuitive feelings last night. I

want to cry. No man has ever said something about baby

making to me and left with feeling warm about it. I heard lovers

in the past say words like baby or marriage and I would cringe

inside. Simply those characters were not for me. Yet maybe

the reality of this, "Want to make a baby" statement, meant I

actually needed to Birth a part of myself I have not let light touch before, and that involved me researching what wants out

of me unto this beautiful dream world without anybody else

suggestion?

I am 28. I am the biggest I have ever been in weight and girth.

I am not pregnant, but in my weight gain I have sometimes

fantasized that I am a mother and that is why I am shaped like

this. It is a strange psychological shift to experience,

especially as a woman who is still discovering her freedom and

gifts she wants to share. I think being a Mother ultimately is a

huge job and I am still trying to nurture myself into wholeness

and bliss. Having a lovely new (boyfriend) Love is spectacular and something I have longed for, so I am extremely thankful for

this new life with him just as it is. And I see in society having a

baby is a metaphor. It is rare a baby is seen for its real

essence or message, unless the family is pure hearted and lays

no insecure projections upon the child. But what is this

symbolic metaphor really expressing?

However it goes woman, always check in with yourself before

making a child outside of yourself. Make sure the child inside

You is Happy and whole. Plus most men make a fine child,

because they need nurturance from a woman just like a baby

does. They need to suck on your breast, be cradled, kissed

tenderly and told how sweet they are as you encourage them to cry. I like taking care of my lover if he is being open and honest with his feelings, because then I see my love and acceptance helps him love and accept himself. And when someone male or female loves and accepts themselves as they are, They can do wonderful amazing things in the universe and really shine their light*However I caution to the excessive needy types who are always crying and need your empathy, because you can become a crutch to them owning their own emotions and taking responsibly for their own. Real Love ultimately wants everyone to grow into who they are in full

acceptance as they are.

Imagine that you have always had someone, a man and a

woman in your life telling you, " You are so unique and amazing

and everything you love blesses you and this world, so always

do what you Love Dear, Always dream your dream into

vision." How does that feel? It may feel like you can finally let

go of everything you are not and fully embrace who you are in

all your beauty and grace. However we each must learn to be

are own Mother and Father who encourages are own

authenticity and true calling in life. Ultimately if you don't have a great Mother or Father, the universe is inviting you to

be your own, and that is So.... much more freeing, than

idealizing your parents and trying to live out "their" dreams for

them. You got your own dreams calling you.

~Money comes, Money goes, But what you love is what

you must Sow~ And what you are is the gold, you are the

gold.~ You can not travel well with weight, But you can travel

great distances with light.~ If you and your heart had a

conversation, what do you think your heart will love to do with

you in this life?~ To master material living U must first master

the spiritual.~ To live in wealth truly, you must live from your faith and calling.~ If you are called, You are the richest of all if you forever answer the call.~People will forget how much money you borrowed. But people will always remember how loving and alive you are and how you inspired them in their own lives.~ Being honest starts with yourself and then letting others know what you discovered is a great way of sharing this truth.~ I will love to be on my path without fear, guilt or shame. I will love to feel Yes to my life I am choosing to live Dreamfully. When you choose your life, even with all its struggles and glories, you are empowering your existence and healing others to do the same. You can go across the universe and see All.. the Sad People dead in a job for money. Don't

let that be you. For that is one of the greatest illusions here

to break open. You are not a slave. You are an evolution. If

you do not do what you don't care for in your heart, you will

be happier and others will be happier to be around you.

~ Keep to your word, But most importantly keep to your

heart's truth and Ultimately you have kept to both your word

and your truth.~ Time is unique in the essence that it records

how long we have been loving. Space is how I make my day.

The canvas is for me to paint my picture of my love in the

universe. We must remember The Dream is what we create

and believe individually.

~ The Arching Wemoon~

I don't know, these tears are of desire. What is it, my lover

wants a child, but not marriage? He has already done that

road with someone else. I have not. I look for security, I long

for its stability in my life. I can and will continue, but I must be

in a solid partnership with my great lover. I have been left

empty so many times. On stage as a performer I would play my

music, and feel empty and lonely. No one understood my

message so far, or maybe they did, but I was not fulfilled from it. I found myself longing for a true friend after every high time

of doing a show or performing my story and songs. Why didn't

I have both glories of performing my music and being

showered with love by my lover afterwards? When do I get

that glory of my dream? To be with Arle makes me want to be

totally loved and supported by him Musically and Artistically

as I'am. I need to hear him say, " I Believe in You and Your

Music and I know that is your path and it will bring you wealth

and fulfillment and I will Love and support you in everyday you

need and want to live out your dream life and calling and

powers, You are a healer by being You, you liberate ALot of

Beings and Souls. I love U*¹¹

Hmm... Did I get it right to have Arle say all this to me, will it

cure me of my ache? No, even if he said it, it means nothing if I

don't believe it. So wishing for words from another s mouth is

really just wishing to say it to yourself and get on with it, your

love. Or what is it That I must put together to Understand

my life Now and Always? Life being a mystery has less need

for this kind of clarity. With Love and Best Regards~The

Vajj

Notes on The Vajj Wemoon Lifestyle

~ All must take a shower before they touch the flower.

~Nothing lasts forever but energy remains.

~Create a garden and nourish it with all you are inside and

out.

~Do not be bogged down by others projections. Simply tell

them who you are, and if you can't tell them just show yourself

the door.

*The ingredients of a Happy yoni are simple, to the root, and

Full of nutrition! I will list a few here to inspire your meals and

simple health* Enjoy burdock root, coconut oil, plain yogurt with wild berries, turmeric, dill, mushrooms, dark chocolate no

sugar, grapefruits, salad greens, olive oil, flax, chia, cherry &

beet juices, apple juice, peppermint tea with rosehips, ginger,

fish oil, arugula, watermelons, fresh water, coconut water and

lots of quiet self love rituals by candle light and moon light.

Enjoy your yoga flow*

There is no need to react to others. It is better to just be

accepting of where you are in each moment. Forget demands,

Do things on your time~ I'm Done reacting to people in

emotional emergency mode, I rather savor my flavor and do

what feels honest. This way what is important will get done

when it is supposed too and with natural divine flow. Simple I

listen*

*Aye Vu.. Why don't you sing me a song... A vu.. why don't

you sing me a song....

Never use Tampons. Let her Drain & flow~ Know your

chemistry and keep sacred connection to your yoni's rhythms.

Sometimes it is necessary to fast and eat no sugar or gluten.

Take time for yourself, even if you are in love and want to

spend your days with your lover, give yourself space. Your

body as a woman can act like a sponge around others and it is good to get clear of everybody else's energy and just be you with you. No body is perfect even if they are your soul mate. Make space and allow yourself to relax from the high intensity of relationship. If your body is acting out of balance, consider your solitude your time to realign with your divine essence and wholeness and strengthen your body and let go of what is No longer serving you, whether it be a person, food item, beverage, drug, or drink. Step into your power and change into your best self now. Reflect on why you are doing what you are doing and visualize changing those habits or ways so that your path is clear to your best self. Also Minimize. Get

rid of stuff and just keep a Few Precious Things. Stuff is

anything you look at that makes you go " Urgh.." So just let it

go and say Yay! I am a simple Happy Abundant Wemoon. I

am most happy being and doing what I love.

Forgiveness~ Yourself and all others Move on and

transcend the lessons of the past into you being a bright

beautiful woman now* For example you know more than ever

because you stopped yoga and you missed it so, now your

teaching it, and that band you gave up, you now have your

own successful solo career in the music arts & inspiration

world, and that food you kept chasing for a fix until it finally

chased you away, and now you eat mostly organic whole

foods, fruits & vegetables, and that sport you stopped due to

thinking your sexy body is permeant, you now walk/run

everyday & lift weights, and that indoor living in a tiny studio

with no bathroom, you now shower outdoors under the stars

and in the greenery of nature and with a happy smile on your

face, and that boyfriend who took you for granted, now you

have a lover who cherishes you and does everything he can to

bring you joy and steadiness, and that woman & man you

always admire, now you have become both of them in all

magnificence* So take your experiences in stride, for it has

brought you to where you are today, more whole, more loving,

more involved* Ahman!

*Hmm... Yoni Dreads, Irritations, Yeasty infections. Calling

you to Heal Up*

Just writing the words can make me cringe. I am no stranger to

the symptoms, but I know I can heal them. Most reactions in

the body root from an emotional belief or feeling. Usually a

mood occurs before an event. Such as being happy to be on

your moon time and taking care of yourself more carefully

because your body wants nurturance and tenderness. Or

feeling excited because you are about to begin taking steps

toward a long held dream. The flow changes when we feel any

emotion at all. So if emotions are taking you on a roller

coaster ride, it may be time to take a space to yourself, breath

in well and listen to what is going on. Remember you are your

lifetime best friend, so you will make resolve if you take the

space to heal yourself and you your best friend (yoni) are

willing. Feelings are guides that tell us Yes go there or No I

don't want to go there. Early I mentioned herbal teas that are

good for yoni balance and rituals to do alone with yourself in nature. However if something is really out of order in your body, it is best to seek help from a Doctor. Online you can google naturopathic doctors or naturopathic cures for finding solutions to your symptoms. A lot of times you will find you can make at home remedies to heal your imbalance.

The dreamer changes~ Be willing to accept life is an ongoing learning & sharing process. Yet underneath everything you already are what you seek. So coming from a whole place it is wise to ask yourself. What it is it that I want to discover next? Ask and you shall receive the answer. For example I have spent the last 4 years exploring my music calling and path and now I feel drawn to other ways of living. I have met a few

doctors lately and I am drawn to the Holistic Health Doctor

path. I have began to research what school will best serve my

interest and goals on this path. I am beginning to get excited

about this new chosen field of study and mastery. It is costly

money wise, but the advantage of having a foundation in my

new chosen interest will help me along this path. Being around

people that share a common goal and interest with me is

powerful and sustaining and I recommend everyone finds some

kind of community to share with and grow your light with. I

have worked in the health food industry for over 10 years

along with studying and teaching yoga, ayurveda, natural

medicine, and spiritual health and healing. So to take the next

step as investing in myself and school feels right. I feel more

ready for this commitment than ever before because I am now

feeling called to this path. No not for the money of being a

doctor, but for the aim of helping others heal themselves

naturally and affectively. It is fun to me to see others reap the

rewards of my universal knowledge and find power within

themselves through my initiation. I am drawn to utilizing my

intuitive healing skills always. Music for instance is my first

calling and I love it dearly and it shows. I have found ways through my music touring and street busking to uplift and

inspire loads of humans* Music is natural to me in my design.

In a way I have been a musical doctor forever and now I am

looking at becoming another kind of doctor utilizes

Aromatherapy, Herbology, Astrology and Spirituality.

However this is all still connected to who I naturally am and

what I am called to do, so it works for me. So I suggest when

you look at becoming anything else than what you already are,

make sure it is complimenting what you naturally possess and

you will Guaranteed be happy with how you are living your life

and dreams to the fullest*

Here is some more inspirations from me to U

~A good challenge is one that enhances you for you in the universe*

~ The better and clearer the goal, the better and happier result*

~Nothing you do pleases anyone, and even though it does, never do it for anyone but you.

~ Forget perfectness, religious ideas, codes of honor, pedastils and separatism, and just be yourself fully.

~You may think God doesn't do that, why do I, Well because you are you*

~Start with your personal child's dream and keep at it till it

sings and keep at it till your heart's content and rewards

exceed your needs and wants.

~ What works is best. What doesn't work is not worth your

precious time and space.

~ Did you really come this far to go hide in a closet? No way,

show the way of your light and don't delay.

~ Try on those shiney shoes you always loved but felt

ashamed about because they were just so... expensive. You

don't have to buy them to enjoy trying them.

~Sing, act, dance, play and then be serious, focused, and on your way, and again Sing, dance, act, and play seriously This is the way*

~ Make the most of what you have for you have everything you want and need to live your life*

~ Notice in detail what you are experiencing Now, and then you shall see you are living your dreams that once longed to come about.

~ If your boyfriend is rich, enjoy the fruits of his generosity freely and gratefully. And when you are rich do the same for him. Because obviously you are on your way to being rich and that is why you are with someone who can teach you about the

quality of generosity richness can have.

~Remember that you are here on your own journey and

callings and you will meet lots of friends along your chosen

path to uplift, love, and support you always and keep you in

tune to U in the Universe*<>

~ MASSAGE YOURSELF~ Heal your Imbalance~

Self pleasuring can equal self mastery. This I know is the key

to yoni health. If you can attune yourself to a loving healing

song and pleasure yourself, you are in for blessings and

equilibrium. Sometimes I cry after a session with myself because I am so happy to reconnect with my essence alone as I am. It is amazing the transformation a magnificent self pleasuring session can bring. Give yourself space, comfort, security, and satisfaction. Set the candles, draw the curtains, play the music and see yourself to joy. I believe you know when you have mastered your own touch because you will no longer seek others for pleasure, you will seek others for fun and learning something new, why else bother with a sexual relationship only, when you know you can totally supply yourself and not risk your body temple to pregnancy or imbalance. I find that I enjoy my boyfriend more when I know I

am acting out of love not desire, not that he can't satisfy me

with his loving energy, but that I prefer to not have that as the

goal in relationship. The relationship feels a lot more free and

kind when you tell your boyfriend I love having you has a great

friend the most. We are responsible only for ourselves and

when we remember this, we can dance so much more joyously

together and alone. I find myself telling my partner what to do.

That is a trap. Do not waist your energy telling another

where they need fixing, instead take their issue as a lesson

that you will not do that to yourself. Such as if they over eat.

Inside say " Thank you for teaching me not to over eat or eat

bad food. And the more you just be you in your self the

better everyone will find their health.

~Cotton Clothes & The Good Products~

Panty free zone. Yes there is no need to wear underwear,

unless you have too. But air flow is essential ya know, breath

is life.

OM and breath many deep relaxed cycles while placing (

cupping) the right hand over your yoni and one hand over

your heart. Also place one hand on your belly button area

and one hand on your heart and or yoni. This tones your

body to its natural peaceful frequency. If you have a partner,

you can ask them to OM with their mouth open & sealed on

top of your yoni, they can OM several times as you breath

deeply and let the frequency radiate through you. Very

pleasing and unique experience here. O

Ocean water is grand. If you live near the sea take a nice 20

minute soak to absorb loads of powerful minerals and

nutrients into your skin. Ocean water is very simular ph to the

yoni naturally, so it will restore your bodies ph just by

swimming in it.

Think god thoughts about yourself and be gentle with your

journey. Shame is an old fashioned way of control and fear

and no body needs or wants that.

Keep a journal. What you are experiencing in life is very

important and special to only you. Nobody gets your

experience but you. So keep a journal and reflect on what

you felt and when with as much detail. A journal will help you

track any habits around your actions made individually and in

regards to your relationships and environments you go to. A

journal can also be full of what you want to create and all the inspiration you feel in life and help guide you more so on your path.

Avoid perfumes and chemicals. Firstly they give you headaches by messing up your hormone system, second they pollute the air, and third they kill you. Find 100% natural essential oils and pure crystal deodorant at health food stores.

Protect yourself. Utilize condoms, especially if you or your partner has had other partners and doesn't know their std's tested status. It is actually quite simple and wise to go get tested and take your new partner with you and Realize it is very easy to be loyal to your health. We are humans in these

body temples and we are magical and earthly and learning

about life. There are free testing places everywhere. Also

you can order std's testing kits online on Amazon.com and

from a local doctor. Yes of course utilize your intuition on

your choice of sexual partners and make your appropriate

action from there. And remember sex with yourself is free of

pregnancy, std's and wtf did I do that for's last night? You

know you don't wake up in question, when you know it was just

you you had last night. You wake up in exuberance and

freedom from making somebody else breakfast*

~MOON, STAR NATURE VISUALIZATION~

You come from a place many have experienced, that may or may not have had human form. You come from a place of purity and light that heals all dimensions of earthly reality. You are a beam of light and your moon, stars, land and sky's embrace your body, laid across this vast earth and energy chamber of gold and evolution robusting. You are sex adequate and beyond measure. You have the freedom to tune yourself home always, the Moon and the stars and the land are just waiting for you to lay your burdens down and open to the frequency of the divine being in which you are. There is no other, the way is through U and your connection to the

here now and beyond Universes.

~ Closing Words~

Welcome to your new relationship with your intuitive divine

self. Keep going from your inspirations and you will surely

enjoy your life. If you read my book and felt things were

missing, email me, tell me what you feel or maybe write your

own story and share your knowledge. We are here to share

are light and the more lights on and shared and blasting in

grace the better* I just wanted to write something simple and

to the point any age girl or woman or male can read and get

understanding and inspiration from about the yoni

uniqueness. Maybe you have never pleasured yourself and

your sex life is shabby, well here you are getting the

encouragement and inspiration to go on and Make Love to U

so that u can Align yourself with your own awesome

frequency and change for the best you. I was 9 when I first

instructed my girlfriends at a sleep over on how to self

pleasure, the mother walked in at my friends and tried to send

me home. Yet then I said to her, " Your a grown woman, don't

you know how to make yourself happy?" She shifted, closed

the door and let us continue. Next week at school my

girlfriends were ecstatic about their own new findings down

there and it was like our sacred little secret, that we as girls

knew how to make ourselves happy, in a world telling us we

needed Ken barbies for husbands to be whole. Ah~ Bullshit!

So wa la* Take yourself home and you might just find exactly

what you've been looking for. Let the art and creation flow~

You might just start drawing lots of flowers in lots of colors*

Enjoy and imagine whatever you want, it is your stage, bring

who ever characters you want and as many as you like. You

may even surprise yourself with what you truly desire in your

design.